I MATTER TOO

90-day Postpartum Gratitude & Self-Care

LISA COLELLA

WWW.THERAINBOWMOM.COM

Dedicated to Kendra & Jada: my greatest teachers and inspirations.
And to all the angels on earth whom someone calls "mom."

ABOUT THERAINBOWMOM.COM

According to my mother, there was a rainbow in the sky when I was born. When she told me this story for the first time, I immediately thought, "it's a sign!" I just didn't know what the meaning of that sign was... Until now.

I'm sure I won't know the full meaning behind that sacred symbol until my life has run its course. But, becoming a mother has certainly brought more clarity about how it relates to my own way of being (and has sparked a desire to share it with others). I have come to realize that I feel more energetic, balanced and connected when I am able to express myself through a spectrum (or rainbow) of identities during any given day, week, or month. In turn, planning for this has helped me navigate the challenging season of young motherhood with a whole lot more presence, patience, and joy than I was able to feel before this revelation.

The term "rainbow mom" is not meant to be an LGBTQ reference, nor is it focused on those who have tragically dealt with the loss of a child (although it is absolutely inclusive of members who identify with either of those communities). It is a symbolic reference to the various identities (or "colors"), through which we express ourselves as wholehearted human beings during any given period of time. It knows no race, age, gender, religion, or other tangible descriptor. Rather, it is a state of mind characterized by a continuous pursuit for more conscious, purposeful and balanced living, to benefit oneself *and* the next generation who follows closely behind.

Furthermore, "rainbow mom" is a metaphor for the perfectly beautiful, imperfectly constructed beings that we are. It is an acceptance of the fact that we are always navigating shades of our truest colors while never being fully at the beginning or end of our emergence. (As a reformed perfectionist, I am still grappling with that last one!)

It is a belief that, even on our self-judged "worst" days—when it seems to be raining all around us—we are still beautiful to someone, none more than our own children.

And finally, it is a reminder that how you experience a child is always a reflection of you, more than of them. They will trigger your unhealed wounds and shine a floodlight on the most authentic parts of you. Being a "rainbow mom" in this context means being a reflection—a refraction—a dispersion of light for your child(ren) as they navigate the many moments of life. After all, it is *your* colors that provide the strength, the vitality, and the brilliance to bring sun to their rainy moments until they are ready to do so on their own.

TheRainbowMom.com is a platform through which I plan to creatively explore these concepts with little reservation and no expectation. It is intended to be a channel that facilitates my own continuous growth, and in turn supports that of other likeminded mothers. It is a gift I wish to share with all my fellow sisters who are striving to embrace humor after challenges, lessons after mistakes, and joy after rain.

EVERY INTERACTION WITH OUR **CHILDREN** IS A **REFLECTION** OF OUR OWN RELATIONSHIP WITH **OURSELVES.**

— DR. SHEFALI TSABARY

INTRODUCTION

Hi Sister,

Welcome to the first chapter in your postpartum journal, and the next chapter in your life story—motherhood.

Whatever has brought you here to this moment, I encourage you to trust that YOUR journey has unfolded exactly how it was meant to. Cultivating a practice of trust in yourself and acceptance of "what is" (instead of wishing for an "ideal") are quite possibly the greatest weapons you can equip yourself with to navigate the nebulous adventure of parenting.

This journal has been my third baby—created and birthed in sync with my second daughter, Jada. It has helped me weather the newborn days much more gracefully with Jada than I did with my first daughter. It has also helped me establish practices and manifest dreams that will carry our family into a healthy, joy-filled future well beyond the postpartum period. I hope that sharing it will inspire the construction and growth of your family in the making as well.

I created this journal to support myself—and to offer a resource that is contrary to the societal constructs in America that currently favor a "baby first" approach during the postpartum period. When compared to the resources, focus, services and gifts rendered to my babies, I experienced a form of oblivious neglect from my health care providers, social networks, and several relatives.

The baby received several fast and routine check-ups, while I was granted only one check-in appointment at 6 weeks postpartum. Furthermore, the literature given to us at the hospital covered the A-Z's of baby care, but had zero information on how I should deal with severe engorgement, hives triggered by Mast Cell Activation Disorder, mastitis, perineal stitches, drowning night sweats, diastasis recti, prolapsed organs, and a whole host of other unpleasant symptoms that showed up in my body like surprise unwelcomed visitors. Even at Jada's one-month appointment, I remember the Nurse Practitioner looking at my (visibly) bleeding nipples and casually suggesting that I try to add 1-2 more feedings each day so that Jada could incease her [already healthy] percentile numbers.

Visitors tended to gift the babies outfits, books, or stuffed animals that they will never remember, while they barely gave my tired bleeding body a hug or hello. I remember thinking to myself so often, "*I matter too.*"

These examples only scratch the surface of the western world's myopic focus on family care following the birth of a child.

I believe that a mother-first approach benefits everyone. When mom's cup is full, everyone else's is able to be poured into; when it's not, everyone thirsts. This makes sense to me on every dimension: physically, a healthy mom is able to produce needed milk (if breastfeeding), and mentally, she is able to demonstrate more patience with a colicky baby or a partner's shortcomings. Even energetically, the baby is so intrinsically connected to the mother after birth that the mom sets the tone for the baby's brand-new experience in this world. Put simply, taking care of oneself, especially in the fragile postpartum days, cannot be overstated. And since the world around me wasn't helping me in an intentional, focused way when I needed it most, I wanted a repeatable way to give that gift of holistic support to *myself*.

And now to others.

This is the first edition of, what I believe will be, an iterative project. I plan to collect as much feedback as possible and make new editions that support moms around the world more and more during one of the most vulnerable and challenging seasons of their life. I certainly hope it helps *you* as you enter yours.

YOUR WEEKLY PRACTICE

For a long time, I convinced myself that I just didn't have time to plan—that I had to *do* so much, how could I possibly have time to plan for it all too? Moreover, I thought that planning was something you did when there were actions involved, and feelings were just something you were subject to as a result of those actions. Over time, I realized this belief was false. Through great reflection and introspection, I realized that I was most anxious and reactive to situations that I hadn't planned for in advance or had an authentic interest in altogether. I also realized that if I wasn't intentional about *creating* balance, it didn't happen.

I am part of several mother groups and female-oriented communities. Within them, I often hear and observe statements like, "I don't really enjoy being a mom" or "I miss my life before I had kids. I don't think those statements represent the whole truth. In many cases, it's not that they don't like being a mom. It's that they don't like being only "Mom".

Like so many other women, I feel most alive when I am expressing myself in a variety of identities throughout a given week: wife, mother, leader, health advocate, friend, entrepreneur, sister, etc. I think of these identities as color buckets in which I make "time deposits." The goal is to feel like a beautifully balanced rainbow of colors at any given time. Too many deposits in one area will create an imbalance in another. Of course, the realities of life make this an ever-shifting target, where "perfect balance" doesn't exist. But severe imbalances become apparent quite quickly.

This sounds simple enough to manage—until giving birth, when one's identity suddenly feels entirely monopolized by "mother." Furthermore, society reinforces that phenomena as "healthy"; one is seen as a "good" mom if she sacrifices all else for the comfort of her child.

Of course, I'm not saying a child's comfort is not important—it absolutely is. I just think the lens through which society looks to achieve that comfort sustainably is backward. Glennon Doyle rightfully pointed out in her book *Untamed* that women have come to be celebrated when they are "selfless"—that the pinnacle of motherhood is for the mom to lose herself in service to her children, partner, and community. I, like her, disagree. We need to be models, not martyrs, for our children because they are *watching* a heck of a lot more than they are *listening*.

And so, it's important to think about the *combination* of identities that make you a whole person and *plan* to make sufficient deposits in those buckets each week.

The most important identities for me are, in no particular order:

1. Connected Friend
2. Conscious Mother
3. Patient Wife
4. Compassionate Family Member
5. Intentional Health Advocate
6. Inspiring Leader/Entrepreneur
7. Imaginative Creator

Now it's time to define yours!

MY BALANCED WEEK:

Parts of Me to Express So That I Feel Whole

Figure 1. Start by listing the seven most important identities that, when expressed, make you feel balanced and whole—the "colors of your rainbow", if you will.

MY "RAINBOW" SELF

1.

2.

3.

4.

5.

6.

7.

Rewrite each one of these into its own color bucket each week. For each identity, list priority actions, activities, or intentions for the week that allow you to make time deposits into that dimension of yourself in an amount that feels right to you in the present moment. There is no mathematical formula here...no rules that say you need an equal number of actions in all buckets, no "best practice" ratio of identities to priorities, and no expectation that you'll account for every single bucket every week. This is an exercise in creating space for you to get in touch with your higher self and for trusting that your intuition will guide you achieving the main goal during this period of your life, which is a balanced mind, body, and spirit *in this moment.*

That being said, I will share one insight that has fundamentally altered how I experience my life, and it's this:

Happiness = reality – expectations

If you set and expect to do 10 or 20 things in one identity each week, but you realistically can only achieve five, you are setting yourself up to live in chronic disappointment. At the same time, we know that, as human beings, we have a genetically wired need to feel a sense of purpose and significance, so some level of goal-setting is healthy. This practice, managed this way during the postpartum period, will also serve as an important mental health aide for you, to counteract the psychological impact of monotonous and intense newborn care.

Figure 1.

1. Connected Friend

- Extend invite for visit to Mary

- Send birthday gift to Gillian

- Send voice message to check

in with at least 1 friend each day

2. Identity #2

Priority actions, to-do's,

appointments, and/or goals for

the week ahead to express this

valued identity of yours.

Identity #3

Priority actions, to-do's,

appointments, and/or goals for

the week ahead to express this

valued identity of yours.

4. Identity #4

Priority actions, to-do's,

appointments, and/or goals for

the week ahead to express this

valued identity of yours.

5. Identity #5

Priority actions, to-do's,

appointments, and/or goals for

the week ahead to express this

valued identity of yours.

6. Identity #6

Priority actions, to-do's,

appointments, and/or goals for

the week ahead to express this

valued identity of yours.

7. Identity #7

Priority actions, to-do's,

appointments, and/or goals for

the week ahead to express this

valued identity of yours.

Figure 2. Reflect on and evaluate your intentions vs. reality from the previous week.

Do a very simple check-in with yourself prior to making your plan for the new week. It's critical that you approach this exercise through the lens of reflection and desire for continuous learning and growth—not for the purpose of self-criticism or blame. The actual outcome is not as important as the way you *feel* about that outcome. The way you feel about it is all the information you'll need to make *the next best move* forward. If you aren't happy with it, make a change. If you are happy with it, have a mini celebration with yourself and build on that success!

So, be real but be graceful when thinking about how well you realized each of your priority intentions:

a.   + = Nailed it
b.   **n** = Neither good nor bad (or maybe a mixture of both)
c.   - = Didn't go so well (there is a learning to take forward into next week)

That's it! You've put intention into your week, which is something that few others do—WELL DONE!

Having this weekly practice made all the difference for me in my second postpartum period. Even when the COVID-19 crisis hit and resulted in us not being able to leave the house or have access to many of the self-care channels I had come to rely on (gyms, chiropractors, etc.), I found ways to make deposits in many identity buckets each week within the home environment I was confined to.

For me, Sundays felt like the most natural day to complete this exercise. It was a perfect grounding point in the week's cycle—a natural point of pause to reflect on the week prior, and a peaceful time to plan for the week ahead. For you, a different day of the week might feel better. Pick a day that works for you and make this planning and reflection exercise a priority.

Also, feel free to review your answers as much or as little as you need to throughout the week. I find that this practice usually leads to a schedule that creates the reality I want to experience. I very rarely need to go back and remind myself of every little detail. Other people may find it useful to do a "refresh" or to check-in periodically throughout the week if things start to feel out of balance. You do you.

Figure 2.

Reflections (from last week)		
Identity	Net Outcome (+ / n / −)	Learnings to take forward
1. Connected Friend	—	Send check-in messages in the morning instead of waiting until evening (witching hour!)
2.		
3.		
4.		
5.		
6.		
7.		

DAILY PRACTICE

In my adult years, specifically since having children, I've come to realize that two things set the tone for the day: 1) how "grounded" mommy is and 2) how she begins the day because, refer to #1. This short, 8-question daily practice is designed to help you ground and set intentions at the beginning of each day as a form of self-care. This will likely help you feel better and will improve your energy levels throughout the day, while also having a positive ripple effect on your entire family.

Your answers don't need to be long, but they should be intentional. They should also be birthed from a place inside your authentic self—not intellectually manufactured from your societally tamed mind. I find that being in a quiet place, alone, with something warm to drink and to wear is key to facilitating access to the deeper parts of my being. Over time, you'll figure out what elements you need to access yours.

The following descriptions provide context behind each prompt question. For maximum effect, review these as needed to ensure you are speaking to the essence of each question, as each has been designed to support a specific part of your mind, body, or spirit during the postpartum period.

Right now, in this moment, I am grateful for...

Time is warped when you have young kids. In some ways, the weeks fly by, but often minutes feel like years when you are having undesirable experiences. Trying to comprehend time during this period in your life is like trying to cage a cloud. During the times I'm flailing in this conundrum, the best thing I can do is to focus on the present moment. My mantra during anxious times is, "In this moment, I am okay." Similarly, answering this question is a chance for you to be in the present moment each morning by focusing on three things (or more) that you are grateful for. They can be big things (like the breathing human being you've just created from scratch) or little things (like the feel of soft slippers on your feet). What matters is that you are forcing your brain to focus on the positive and are priming it to look for things to be grateful for throughout the day. After all, you'll be asked the same question tomorrow!

The MOST important thing I can do to feel good about myself today is...

Anything is better than nothing. This is not a time to think about what you should say in response to this question. It's an invitation to go inward into your own body, mind, and spirit and deliver joy to the place that needs it most. Because let's be honest, no one else is thinking about your well-being as deeply or as thoughtfully, and you deserve to feel good more than you ever have before. It is by answering this question that I discovered how everyday things can be luxuries when I view them as such, especially when I only have time for one or two while caring for a helpless human being. Some days I needed to do my makeup to feel human, other days I needed to make my favorite smoothie a non-negotiable, and other days I needed to look at old travel pictures to remind myself that there was still a world outside my house ready to embrace me with open arms when I was done wrapping my arms around my newest wonder. I never would have prioritized these lifesaving agenda items if I hadn't asked myself this question explicitly every day.

Today, I want to be...

Be intentional when answering this question. Close your eyes and envision the presence you want to have with your family, with your friends, and with yourself. Think about the story you want to tell about yourself a week, a month, or a year from now and describe what that looks like for your being today.

Do you want to be the wounded child or flailing adolescent of your past? Or do you want to be the strong and inspiring adult you are today? Do you want to challenge yourself to be patient in times of stress? Or be an extra-loving spouse to a partner who is struggling with this life transition? Translate who you aspire to be into a way of being today, and then watch yourself live into it!

Today, I want to feel...

You get to choose. If there is one thing my 2 ½-year-old daughter knows about mornings at our house, it is that I will be asking her the question, "How do you want to feel today?" within 10 minutes of our first morning hug. It is important to me that she grow up knowing that she gets to choose how she feels each day, each hour, each moment. Life, her ego, her friends, and so many other forces will deliver "suggestions" to her psyche, but only she has the ability to decide what suggestions she will accept and which ones she will reject or let go of. And so, it's important that you feel that same empowerment when starting your day. There can be dozens of reasons (physiologically, practically, and emotionally) to feel frustrated, sad, depressed, disheartened, angry, impatient, tired, and so on after having a baby. Choose joy (or whatever it is you wish to feel) instead, and experience the ordinary as extraordinary.

I am so much stronger than...

Whatever it is your body, mind, or spirit is experiencing as challenges today—whatever barriers are keeping you from achieving the state of being and feeling you've noted above, affirm your strength over them here. During my postpartum journey, my answers to this prompt ranged from "this unknown, itchy rash" to "these feelings of sadness" to "my bleeding nipples" to "exhaustion." This is not the time to judge yourself; this is the time to be your own number one fan and know that your higher self is bigger than any challenge, and stronger than any form of pain you're experiencing. Once your mind is convinced that it will heal, your body will catch up.

Today's headline: _____

Pretend you are a journalist and will be capturing the MOST important part of your day's experience in one single headline. What would you want it to be? A friend shared the following anecdote on social media during the 2020 global COVID-19 pandemic. I think it is a beautiful description of what this prompt is designed to help you achieve—a reminder that you can consume news, but choose to create your own headlines that fill your headspace and heart space with positivity if you don't like the external perspective:

Sometimes I just want to stop. Talk of COVID, protests, looting, brutality. I lose my way. Become convinced that this "new normal is real life.

But then I meet an 87-year old who talks of living through Polio, diphtheria, Vietnam protests, and yet is still enchanted with life. He seemed surprised when I said that 2020 must be especially challenging for him. "No", he said slowly looking me straight in the eyes, "I learned a long time ago to not see the world through the printed headlines. I see the world through the people that surround me. I see the world with realization that we love big. Therefore, I just choose to write my own headlines...

"Husband Loves Wife Today."

"Family Drops Everything to Come to Grandma's Bedside."

He patted my hand, *"Old Man Makes New Friend."*

His words collide with my worries, freeing them from the tether I had been holding tight. They float away, and I am left with a renewed spirit. My headline now reads, *"Woman Overwhelmed by the Spirit of Kindness and the Reminder that the Capacity to Love is Never-ending."*

One dream I have for my family in five years is...

Uncage your imagination and let it run wild with this one! As mentioned, time has a way of slowing down in the day-to-day chess game of having young kids. The daunting black hole of isolation can falsely whisper "this is forever" during the monotonous responsibilities, often creating a dense fog that hides the beauty of today and the exciting dreams of tomorrow from your higher self. As a dreamer and creator, this proved to be such an important question to ponder in my postpartum journey. It ignited my creative spirit and gave me a daily reminder of my "why." It also gave me the relief I was often grasping for, knowing that all the hard parts were just part of the journey and would prove to be worth it for years to come. Sometimes our imagination is the greatest escape from the challenges of today.

That's it, my friend!

Now it's time to dive in, take care of yourself, and let the rest fall as it may. I hope you experience a wholehearted journey filled with an abundance of love, healing, and strength.

IN A SOCIETY THAT SAYS,
"PUT YOURSELF LAST,"
SELF-LOVE AND
SELF-ACCEPTANCE
ARE ALMOST
REVOLUTIONARY.

– BRENÉ BROWN

Week 1: __ / __ / __

Right now, in this moment, I am grateful for...

_____

_____

_____

_____

The MOST important thing I can do to feel good about myself today is...

_____

_____

_____

Today, I want to be...

_____

_____

_____

_____

_____

_____

_____

_____

_____

Today, I want to feel...

_____
_____
_____
_____

I am so much stronger than...

_____
_____
_____
_____

Today's headline:

_____
_____

One dream I have for my family in five years is...

_____
_____
_____
_____
_____

Right now, in this moment, I am grateful for...

_____

_____

_____

_____

The MOST important thing I can do to feel good about myself today is...

_____

_____

_____

Today, I want to be...

_____

_____

_____

_____

_____

_____

_____

_____

Today, I want to feel...

_____

_____

_____

_____

I am so much stronger than...

_____

_____

_____

_____

Today's headline:

_____

_____

One dream I have for my family in five years is...

_____

_____

_____

_____

_____

Right now, in this moment, I am grateful for...

_____
_____
_____
_____

The MOST important thing I can do to feel good about myself today is...

_____
_____
_____

Today, I want to be...

_____
_____
_____
_____
_____
_____
_____
_____

Today, I want to feel...

_____

_____

_____

_____

I am so much stronger than...

_____

_____

_____

_____

Today's headline:

_____

_____

One dream I have for my family in five years is...

_____

_____

_____

_____

_____

Week 1, Day 4

Right now, in this moment, I am grateful for...

_____
_____
_____
_____

The MOST important thing I can do to feel good about myself today is...

_____
_____
_____

Today, I want to be...

_____
_____
_____
_____
_____
_____
_____
_____
_____

Today, I want to feel…

I am so much stronger than…

Today's headline:

One dream I have for my family in five years is…

Right now, in this moment, I am grateful for...

_____

_____

_____

_____

The MOST important thing I can do to feel good about myself today is...

_____

_____

_____

Today, I want to be...

_____

_____

_____

_____

_____

_____

_____

_____

Today, I want to feel...

_____

_____

_____

_____

I am so much stronger than...

_____

_____

_____

_____

Today's headline:

_____

_____

One dream I have for my family in five years is...

_____

_____

_____

_____

_____

Week 1, Day 6

Right now, in this moment, I am grateful for...

_____

_____

_____

_____

The MOST important thing I can do to feel good about myself today is...

_____

_____

_____

Today, I want to be...

_____

_____

_____

_____

_____

_____

_____

_____

_____

Today, I want to feel...

_____

_____

_____

_____

I am so much stronger than...

_____

_____

_____

_____

Today's headline:

_____

_____

One dream I have for my family in five years is...

_____

_____

_____

_____

_____

Right now, in this moment, I am grateful for...

_____

_____

_____

_____

The MOST important thing I can do to feel good about myself today is...

_____

_____

_____

Today, I want to be...

_____

_____

_____

_____

_____

_____

_____

_____

_____

Today, I want to feel…

_____

_____

_____

_____

I am so much stronger than…

_____

_____

_____

_____

Today's headline:

_____

_____

One dream I have for my family in five years is…

_____

_____

_____

_____

_____

	Reflections (from last week)		
	Identity	Net Outcome $(+ / n / -)$	Learnings to take forward
1.			
2.			
3.			
4.			
5.			
6.			
7.			

Week 2: __ / __ / __

Right now, in this moment, I am grateful for...

_____

_____

_____

_____

The MOST important thing I can do to feel good about myself today is...

_____

_____

_____

Today, I want to be...

_____

_____

_____

_____

_____

_____

_____

_____

_____

Today, I want to feel…

_____

_____

_____

_____

I am so much stronger than…

_____

_____

_____

_____

Today's headline:

_____

_____

One dream I have for my family in five years is…

_____

_____

_____

_____

_____

Right now, in this moment, I am grateful for...

_____

_____

_____

_____

The MOST important thing I can do to feel good about myself today is...

_____

_____

_____

Today, I want to be...

_____

_____

_____

_____

_____

_____

_____

_____

_____

Today, I want to feel...

_____

_____

_____

_____

I am so much stronger than...

_____

_____

_____

_____

Today's headline:

_____

_____

One dream I have for my family in five years is...

_____

_____

_____

_____

_____

Right now, in this moment, I am grateful for...

_____

_____

_____

_____

The MOST important thing I can do to feel good about myself today is...

_____

_____

_____

Today, I want to be...

_____

_____

_____

_____

_____

_____

_____

_____

_____

Today, I want to feel...

_____

_____

_____

_____

I am so much stronger than...

_____

_____

_____

_____

Today's headline:

_____

_____

One dream I have for my family in five years is...

_____

_____

_____

_____

_____

Right now, in this moment, I am grateful for...

_____

_____

_____

_____

The MOST important thing I can do to feel good about myself today is...

_____

_____

_____

Today, I want to be...

_____

_____

_____

_____

_____

_____

_____

_____

_____

Today, I want to feel...

_____

_____

_____

_____

I am so much stronger than...

_____

_____

_____

_____

Today's headline:

_____

_____

One dream I have for my family in five years is...

_____

_____

_____

_____

_____

Right now, in this moment, I am grateful for...

_____

_____

_____

_____

The MOST important thing I can do to feel good about myself today is...

_____

_____

_____

Today, I want to be...

_____

_____

_____

_____

_____

_____

_____

_____

_____

Today, I want to feel...

_____

_____

_____

_____

I am so much stronger than...

_____

_____

_____

_____

Today's headline:

_____

_____

One dream I have for my family in five years is...

_____

_____

_____

_____

_____

Right now, in this moment, I am grateful for...

_____

_____

_____

_____

The MOST important thing I can do to feel good about myself today is...

_____

_____

_____

Today, I want to be...

_____

_____

_____

_____

_____

_____

_____

_____

_____

Today, I want to feel...

_____

_____

_____

_____

I am so much stronger than...

_____

_____

_____

_____

Today's headline:

_____

_____

One dream I have for my family in five years is...

_____

_____

_____

_____

_____

Right now, in this moment, I am grateful for...

_____

_____

_____

_____

The MOST important thing I can do to feel good about myself today is...

_____

_____

_____

Today, I want to be...

_____

_____

_____

_____

_____

_____

_____

_____

_____

Today, I want to feel...

_____

_____

_____

_____

I am so much stronger than...

_____

_____

_____

_____

Today's headline:

_____

_____

One dream I have for my family in five years is...

_____

_____

_____

_____

_____

	Reflections (from last week)	
Identity	Net Outcome (+ / n / −)	Learnings to take forward
1.		
2.		
3.		
4.		
5.		
6.		
7.		

Week 3: __ / __ / __

Right now, in this moment, I am grateful for...

_____

_____

_____

_____

The MOST important thing I can do to feel good about myself today is...

_____

_____

_____

Today, I want to be...

_____

_____

_____

_____

_____

_____

_____

_____

_____

Today, I want to feel…

_____

_____

_____

_____

I am so much stronger than…

_____

_____

_____

_____

Today's headline:

_____

_____

One dream I have for my family in five years is…

_____

_____

_____

_____

_____

Right now, in this moment, I am grateful for...

_____

_____

_____

_____

The MOST important thing I can do to feel good about myself today is...

_____

_____

_____

Today, I want to be...

_____

_____

_____

_____

_____

_____

_____

_____

_____

Today, I want to feel...

_____

_____

_____

_____

I am so much stronger than...

_____

_____

_____

_____

Today's headline:

_____

_____

One dream I have for my family in five years is...

_____

_____

_____

_____

_____

Right now, in this moment, I am grateful for...

_____

_____

_____

_____

The MOST important thing I can do to feel good about myself today is...

_____

_____

_____

Today, I want to be...

_____

_____

_____

_____

_____

_____

_____

_____

_____

Today, I want to feel...

_____

_____

_____

_____

I am so much stronger than...

_____

_____

_____

_____

Today's headline:

_____

_____

One dream I have for my family in five years is...

_____

_____

_____

_____

_____

Right now, in this moment, I am grateful for...

_____

_____

_____

_____

The MOST important thing I can do to feel good about myself today is...

_____

_____

_____

Today, I want to be...

_____

_____

_____

_____

_____

_____

_____

_____

_____

Today, I want to feel…

_____

_____

_____

_____

I am so much stronger than…

_____

_____

_____

_____

Today's headline:

_____

_____

One dream I have for my family in five years is…

_____

_____

_____

_____

_____

Right now, in this moment, I am grateful for...

_____

_____

_____

_____

The MOST important thing I can do to feel good about myself today is...

_____

_____

_____

Today, I want to be...

_____

_____

_____

_____

_____

_____

_____

_____

_____

Today, I want to feel...

_____

_____

_____

_____

I am so much stronger than...

_____

_____

_____

_____

Today's headline:

_____

_____

One dream I have for my family in five years is...

_____

_____

_____

_____

_____

Right now, in this moment, I am grateful for...

_____

_____

_____

_____

The MOST important thing I can do to feel good about myself today is...

_____

_____

_____

Today, I want to be...

_____

_____

_____

_____

_____

_____

_____

_____

_____

Today, I want to feel…

I am so much stronger than…

Today's headline:

One dream I have for my family in five years is…

Week 3, Day 7

Right now, in this moment, I am grateful for...

_____
_____
_____
_____

The MOST important thing I can do to feel good about myself today is...

_____
_____
_____

Today, I want to be...

_____
_____
_____
_____
_____
_____
_____
_____
_____

Today, I want to feel...

_____

_____

_____

_____

I am so much stronger than...

_____

_____

_____

_____

Today's headline:

_____

_____

One dream I have for my family in five years is...

_____

_____

_____

_____

_____

	Reflections (from last week)		
	Identity	Net Outcome (+ / n / −)	Learnings to take forward
1.			
2.			
3.			
4.			
5.			
6.			
7.			

Right now, in this moment, I am grateful for...

_____

_____

_____

_____

The MOST important thing I can do to feel good about myself today is...

_____

_____

_____

Today, I want to be...

_____

_____

_____

_____

_____

_____

_____

_____

_____

Today, I want to feel...

_____

_____

_____

_____

I am so much stronger than...

_____

_____

_____

_____

Today's headline:

_____

_____

One dream I have for my family in five years is...

_____

_____

_____

_____

_____

Right now, in this moment, I am grateful for...

The MOST important thing I can do to feel good about myself today is...

Today, I want to be...

Today, I want to feel...

_____

_____

_____

_____

I am so much stronger than...

_____

_____

_____

_____

Today's headline:

_____

_____

One dream I have for my family in five years is...

_____

_____

_____

_____

_____

Right now, in this moment, I am grateful for...

_____

_____

_____

_____

The MOST important thing I can do to feel good about myself today is...

_____

_____

_____

Today, I want to be...

_____

_____

_____

_____

_____

_____

_____

_____

_____

Today, I want to feel...

_____

_____

_____

_____

I am so much stronger than...

_____

_____

_____

_____

Today's headline:

_____

_____

One dream I have for my family in five years is...

_____

_____

_____

_____

_____

Right now, in this moment, I am grateful for...

The MOST important thing I can do to feel good about myself today is...

Today, I want to be...

Today, I want to feel…

_____

_____

_____

_____

I am so much stronger than…

_____

_____

_____

_____

Today's headline:

_____

_____

One dream I have for my family in five years is…

_____

_____

_____

_____

_____

Right now, in this moment, I am grateful for...

_____

_____

_____

_____

The MOST important thing I can do to feel good about myself today is...

_____

_____

_____

Today, I want to be...

_____

_____

_____

_____

_____

_____

_____

_____

_____

Today, I want to feel...

_____

_____

_____

_____

I am so much stronger than...

_____

_____

_____

_____

Today's headline:

_____

_____

One dream I have for my family in five years is...

_____

_____

_____

_____

_____

Right now, in this moment, I am grateful for...

_____

_____

_____

_____

The MOST important thing I can do to feel good about myself today is...

_____

_____

_____

Today, I want to be...

_____

_____

_____

_____

_____

_____

_____

_____

_____

Today, I want to feel...

_____

_____

_____

_____

I am so much stronger than...

_____

_____

_____

_____

Today's headline:

_____

_____

One dream I have for my family in five years is...

_____

_____

_____

_____

_____

Right now, in this moment, I am grateful for...

_____

_____

_____

_____

The MOST important thing I can do to feel good about myself today is...

_____

_____

_____

Today, I want to be...

_____

_____

_____

_____

_____

_____

_____

_____

Today, I want to feel…

_____

_____

_____

_____

I am so much stronger than…

_____

_____

_____

_____

Today's headline:

_____

_____

One dream I have for my family in five years is…

_____

_____

_____

_____

_____

Reflections (from last week)		
Identity	Net Outcome (+ / n / −)	Learnings to take forward
1.		
2.		
3.		
4.		
5.		
6.		
7.		

Week 5: __ / __ / __

83

Right now, in this moment, I am grateful for...

_____

_____

_____

_____

The MOST important thing I can do to feel good about myself today is...

_____

_____

_____

Today, I want to be...

_____

_____

_____

_____

_____

_____

_____

_____

_____

Today, I want to feel…

_____

_____

_____

_____

I am so much stronger than…

_____

_____

_____

_____

Today's headline:

_____

_____

One dream I have for my family in five years is…

_____

_____

_____

_____

_____

Right now, in this moment, I am grateful for...

_____

_____

_____

_____

The MOST important thing I can do to feel good about myself today is...

_____

_____

_____

Today, I want to be...

_____

_____

_____

_____

_____

_____

_____

_____

_____

Today, I want to feel...

_____

_____

_____

_____

I am so much stronger than...

_____

_____

_____

_____

Today's headline:

_____

_____

One dream I have for my family in five years is...

_____

_____

_____

_____

_____

Right now, in this moment, I am grateful for...

_____

_____

_____

_____

The MOST important thing I can do to feel good about myself today is...

_____

_____

_____

Today, I want to be...

_____

_____

_____

_____

_____

_____

_____

_____

_____

Today, I want to feel...

_____

_____

_____

_____

I am so much stronger than...

_____

_____

_____

_____

Today's headline:

_____

_____

One dream I have for my family in five years is...

_____

_____

_____

_____

_____

Week 5, Day 4

Right now, in this moment, I am grateful for...

_____

_____

_____

_____

The MOST important thing I can do to feel good about myself today is...

_____

_____

_____

Today, I want to be...

_____

_____

_____

_____

_____

_____

_____

_____

_____

Today, I want to feel...

_____

_____

_____

_____

I am so much stronger than...

_____

_____

_____

_____

Today's headline:

_____

_____

One dream I have for my family in five years is...

_____

_____

_____

_____

_____

Right now, in this moment, I am grateful for…

_____

_____

_____

_____

The MOST important thing I can do to feel good about myself today is…

_____

_____

_____

Today, I want to be…

_____

_____

_____

_____

_____

_____

_____

_____

Today, I want to feel…

_____

_____

_____

_____

I am so much stronger than…

_____

_____

_____

_____

Today's headline:

_____

_____

One dream I have for my family in five years is…

_____

_____

_____

_____

_____

Right now, in this moment, I am grateful for...

_____

_____

_____

_____

The MOST important thing I can do to feel good about myself today is...

_____

_____

_____

Today, I want to be...

_____

_____

_____

_____

_____

_____

_____

_____

_____

Today, I want to feel...

_____

_____

_____

_____

I am so much stronger than...

_____

_____

_____

_____

Today's headline:

_____

_____

One dream I have for my family in five years is...

_____

_____

_____

_____

_____

Right now, in this moment, I am grateful for...

_____
_____
_____
_____

The MOST important thing I can do to feel good about myself today is...

_____
_____
_____

Today, I want to be...

_____
_____
_____
_____
_____
_____
_____
_____
_____

Today, I want to feel...

_____

_____

_____

_____

I am so much stronger than...

_____

_____

_____

_____

Today's headline:

_____

_____

One dream I have for my family in five years is...

_____

_____

_____

_____

_____

	Identity	Net Outcome (+ / n / −)	Learnings to take forward
	Reflections (from last week)		
1.			
2.			
3.			
4.			
5.			
6.			
7.			

Right now, in this moment, I am grateful for...

_____

_____

_____

_____

The MOST important thing I can do to feel good about myself today is...

_____

_____

_____

Today, I want to be...

_____

_____

_____

_____

_____

_____

_____

_____

_____

Today, I want to feel...

_____

_____

_____

_____

I am so much stronger than...

_____

_____

_____

_____

Today's headline:

_____

_____

One dream I have for my family in five years is...

_____

_____

_____

_____

_____

Right now, in this moment, I am grateful for...

_____

_____

_____

_____

The MOST important thing I can do to feel good about myself today is...

_____

_____

_____

Today, I want to be...

_____

_____

_____

_____

_____

_____

_____

_____

_____

Today, I want to feel...

_____

_____

_____

_____

I am so much stronger than...

_____

_____

_____

_____

Today's headline:

_____

_____

One dream I have for my family in five years is...

_____

_____

_____

_____

_____

Week 6, Day 3

Right now, in this moment, I am grateful for...

_____

_____

_____

_____

The MOST important thing I can do to feel good about myself today is...

_____

_____

_____

Today, I want to be...

_____

_____

_____

_____

_____

_____

_____

_____

_____

Today, I want to feel…

_____

_____

_____

_____

I am so much stronger than…

_____

_____

_____

_____

Today's headline:

_____

_____

One dream I have for my family in five years is…

_____

_____

_____

_____

_____

Right now, in this moment, I am grateful for...

_____

_____

_____

_____

The MOST important thing I can do to feel good about myself today is...

_____

_____

_____

Today, I want to be...

_____

_____

_____

_____

_____

_____

_____

_____

_____

Today, I want to feel...

_____

_____

_____

_____

I am so much stronger than...

_____

_____

_____

_____

Today's headline:

_____

_____

One dream I have for my family in five years is...

_____

_____

_____

_____

_____

Right now, in this moment, I am grateful for...

_____

_____

_____

_____

The MOST important thing I can do to feel good about myself today is...

_____

_____

_____

Today, I want to be...

_____

_____

_____

_____

_____

_____

_____

_____

_____

Today, I want to feel...

_____

_____

_____

_____

I am so much stronger than...

_____

_____

_____

_____

Today's headline:

_____

_____

One dream I have for my family in five years is...

_____

_____

_____

_____

_____

Right now, in this moment, I am grateful for...

_____

_____

_____

_____

The MOST important thing I can do to feel good about myself today is...

_____

_____

_____

Today, I want to be...

_____

_____

_____

_____

_____

_____

_____

_____

_____

Today, I want to feel…

_____

_____

_____

_____

I am so much stronger than…

_____

_____

_____

_____

Today's headline:

_____

_____

One dream I have for my family in five years is…

_____

_____

_____

_____

_____

Right now, in this moment, I am grateful for...

_____

_____

_____

_____

The MOST important thing I can do to feel good about myself today is...

_____

_____

_____

Today, I want to be...

_____

_____

_____

_____

_____

_____

_____

_____

_____

_____

Today, I want to feel...

_____
_____
_____
_____

I am so much stronger than...

_____
_____
_____
_____

Today's headline:

_____
_____

One dream I have for my family in five years is...

_____
_____
_____
_____
_____

Week 6: __ / __ / __

	Reflections (from last week)		
	Identity	Net Outcome (+ / n / −)	Learnings to take forward
1.			
2.			
3.			
4.			
5.			
6.			
7.			

Right now, in this moment, I am grateful for...

_____

_____

_____

_____

The MOST important thing I can do to feel good about myself today is...

_____

_____

_____

Today, I want to be...

_____

_____

_____

_____

_____

_____

_____

_____

_____

Today, I want to feel...

_____

_____

_____

_____

I am so much stronger than...

_____

_____

_____

_____

Today's headline:

_____

_____

One dream I have for my family in five years is...

_____

_____

_____

_____

_____

Right now, in this moment, I am grateful for...

_____

_____

_____

_____

The MOST important thing I can do to feel good about myself today is...

_____

_____

_____

Today, I want to be...

_____

_____

_____

_____

_____

_____

_____

_____

_____

Today, I want to feel...

I am so much stronger than...

Today's headline:

One dream I have for my family in five years is...

Right now, in this moment, I am grateful for...

_____

_____

_____

_____

The MOST important thing I can do to feel good about myself today is...

_____

_____

_____

Today, I want to be...

_____

_____

_____

_____

_____

_____

_____

_____

_____

Today, I want to feel…

_____
_____
_____
_____

I am so much stronger than…

_____
_____
_____
_____

Today's headline:

_____
_____

One dream I have for my family in five years is…

_____
_____
_____
_____
_____

Right now, in this moment, I am grateful for...

The MOST important thing I can do to feel good about myself today is...

Today, I want to be...

Today, I want to feel...

_____

_____

_____

_____

I am so much stronger than...

_____

_____

_____

_____

Today's headline:

_____

_____

One dream I have for my family in five years is...

_____

_____

_____

_____

_____

Right now, in this moment, I am grateful for...

_____

_____

_____

_____

The MOST important thing I can do to feel good about myself today is...

_____

_____

_____

Today, I want to be...

_____

_____

_____

_____

_____

_____

_____

_____

_____

Today, I want to feel…

I am so much stronger than…

Today's headline:

One dream I have for my family in five years is…

Right now, in this moment, I am grateful for...

_____

_____

_____

_____

The MOST important thing I can do to feel good about myself today is...

_____

_____

_____

Today, I want to be...

_____

_____

_____

_____

_____

_____

_____

_____

_____

Today, I want to feel...

I am so much stronger than...

Today's headline:

One dream I have for my family in five years is...

Right now, in this moment, I am grateful for…

_____

_____

_____

_____

The MOST important thing I can do to feel good about myself today is…

_____

_____

_____

Today, I want to be…

_____

_____

_____

_____

_____

_____

_____

_____

_____

Today, I want to feel...

_____
_____
_____
_____

I am so much stronger than...

_____
_____
_____
_____

Today's headline:

_____
_____

One dream I have for my family in five years is...

_____
_____
_____
_____
_____

Week 7: __ / __ / __

	Reflections (from last week)		
	Identity	Net Outcome (+ / n / −)	Learnings to take forward
1.			
2.			
3.			
4.			
5.			
6.			
7.			

Right now, in this moment, I am grateful for...

_____

_____

_____

_____

The MOST important thing I can do to feel good about myself today is...

_____

_____

_____

Today, I want to be...

_____

_____

_____

_____

_____

_____

_____

_____

_____

Today, I want to feel…

_____

_____

_____

_____

I am so much stronger than…

_____

_____

_____

_____

Today's headline:

_____

_____

One dream I have for my family in five years is…

_____

_____

_____

_____

_____

Right now, in this moment, I am grateful for...

The MOST important thing I can do to feel good about myself today is...

Today, I want to be...

Today, I want to feel...

_____

_____

_____

_____

I am so much stronger than...

_____

_____

_____

_____

Today's headline:

_____

_____

One dream I have for my family in five years is...

_____

_____

_____

_____

_____

Right now, in this moment, I am grateful for...

_____

_____

_____

_____

The MOST important thing I can do to feel good about myself today is...

_____

_____

_____

Today, I want to be...

_____

_____

_____

_____

_____

_____

_____

_____

_____

_____

Today, I want to feel...

_____
_____
_____
_____

I am so much stronger than...

_____
_____
_____
_____

Today's headline:

_____
_____

One dream I have for my family in five years is...

_____
_____
_____
_____
_____

Right now, in this moment, I am grateful for...

_____

_____

_____

_____

The MOST important thing I can do to feel good about myself today is...

_____

_____

_____

Today, I want to be...

_____

_____

_____

_____

_____

_____

_____

_____

_____

Today, I want to feel...

_____

_____

_____

_____

I am so much stronger than...

_____

_____

_____

_____

Today's headline:

_____

_____

One dream I have for my family in five years is...

_____

_____

_____

_____

_____

Week 7, Day 5

Right now, in this moment, I am grateful for...

_____
_____
_____
_____

The MOST important thing I can do to feel good about myself today is...

_____
_____
_____

Today, I want to be...

_____
_____
_____
_____
_____
_____
_____
_____
_____

Today, I want to feel...

_____

_____

_____

_____

I am so much stronger than...

_____

_____

_____

_____

Today's headline:

_____

_____

One dream I have for my family in five years is...

_____

_____

_____

_____

_____

Right now, in this moment, I am grateful for...

_____

_____

_____

_____

The MOST important thing I can do to feel good about myself today is...

_____

_____

_____

Today, I want to be...

_____

_____

_____

_____

_____

_____

_____

_____

_____

Today, I want to feel...

_____

_____

_____

_____

I am so much stronger than...

_____

_____

_____

_____

Today's headline:

_____

_____

One dream I have for my family in five years is...

_____

_____

_____

_____

_____

Right now, in this moment, I am grateful for...

The MOST important thing I can do to feel good about myself today is...

Today, I want to be...

Today, I want to feel...

_____

_____

_____

_____

I am so much stronger than...

_____

_____

_____

_____

Today's headline:

_____

_____

One dream I have for my family in five years is...

_____

_____

_____

_____

_____

Week 8: __ / __ / __

	Reflections (from last week)		
	Identity	Net Outcome (+ / n / −)	Learnings to take forward
1.			
2.			
3.			
4.			
5.			
6.			
7.			

Right now, in this moment, I am grateful for...

_____
_____
_____
_____

The MOST important thing I can do to feel good about myself today is...

_____
_____
_____

Today, I want to be...

_____
_____
_____
_____
_____
_____
_____
_____
_____

Today, I want to feel...

I am so much stronger than...

Today's headline:

One dream I have for my family in five years is...

Right now, in this moment, I am grateful for...

_____

_____

_____

_____

The MOST important thing I can do to feel good about myself today is...

_____

_____

_____

Today, I want to be...

_____

_____

_____

_____

_____

_____

_____

_____

_____

Today, I want to feel...

_____

_____

_____

_____

I am so much stronger than...

_____

_____

_____

_____

Today's headline:

_____

_____

One dream I have for my family in five years is...

_____

_____

_____

_____

_____

Right now, in this moment, I am grateful for...

The MOST important thing I can do to feel good about myself today is...

Today, I want to be...

Today, I want to feel…

I am so much stronger than…

Today's headline:

One dream I have for my family in five years is…

Right now, in this moment, I am grateful for...

_____

_____

_____

_____

The MOST important thing I can do to feel good about myself today is...

_____

_____

_____

Today, I want to be...

_____

_____

_____

_____

_____

_____

_____

_____

_____

Today, I want to feel…

I am so much stronger than…

Today's headline:

One dream I have for my family in five years is…

Right now, in this moment, I am grateful for...

_____

_____

_____

_____

The MOST important thing I can do to feel good about myself today is...

_____

_____

_____

Today, I want to be...

_____

_____

_____

_____

_____

_____

_____

_____

_____

Week 8, Day 5

Today, I want to feel…

_____
_____
_____
_____

I am so much stronger than…

_____
_____
_____
_____

Today's headline:

_____
_____

One dream I have for my family in five years is…

_____
_____
_____
_____
_____

Right now, in this moment, I am grateful for...

_____

_____

_____

_____

The MOST important thing I can do to feel good about myself today is...

_____

_____

_____

Today, I want to be...

_____

_____

_____

_____

_____

_____

_____

_____

_____

_____

Today, I want to feel...

_____

_____

_____

_____

I am so much stronger than...

_____

_____

_____

_____

Today's headline:

_____

_____

One dream I have for my family in five years is...

_____

_____

_____

_____

_____

Right now, in this moment, I am grateful for...

_____

_____

_____

_____

The MOST important thing I can do to feel good about myself today is...

_____

_____

_____

Today, I want to be...

_____

_____

_____

_____

_____

_____

_____

_____

_____

Today, I want to feel...

_____
_____
_____
_____

I am so much stronger than...

_____
_____
_____
_____

Today's headline:

_____
_____

One dream I have for my family in five years is...

_____
_____
_____
_____
_____

	Reflections (from last week)		
	Identity	Net Outcome (+ / n / −)	Learnings to take forward
1.			
2.			
3.			
4.			
5.			
6.			
7.			

Right now, in this moment, I am grateful for...

_____

_____

_____

_____

The MOST important thing I can do to feel good about myself today is...

_____

_____

_____

Today, I want to be...

_____

_____

_____

_____

_____

_____

_____

_____

_____

Today, I want to feel...

_____

_____

_____

_____

I am so much stronger than...

_____

_____

_____

_____

Today's headline:

_____

_____

One dream I have for my family in five years is...

_____

_____

_____

_____

_____

Right now, in this moment, I am grateful for...

_____

_____

_____

_____

The MOST important thing I can do to feel good about myself today is...

_____

_____

_____

Today, I want to be...

_____

_____

_____

_____

_____

_____

_____

_____

_____

Today, I want to feel…

_____

_____

_____

_____

I am so much stronger than…

_____

_____

_____

_____

Today's headline:

_____

_____

One dream I have for my family in five years is…

_____

_____

_____

_____

_____

Right now, in this moment, I am grateful for...

_____

_____

_____

_____

The MOST important thing I can do to feel good about myself today is...

_____

_____

_____

Today, I want to be...

_____

_____

_____

_____

_____

_____

_____

_____

_____

Today, I want to feel...

_____

_____

_____

_____

I am so much stronger than...

_____

_____

_____

_____

Today's headline:

_____

_____

One dream I have for my family in five years is...

_____

_____

_____

_____

_____

Week 9, Day 4

Right now, in this moment, I am grateful for…

_____
_____
_____
_____

The MOST important thing I can do to feel good about myself today is…

_____
_____
_____

Today, I want to be…

_____
_____
_____
_____
_____
_____
_____
_____

Today, I want to feel...

_____

_____

_____

_____

I am so much stronger than...

_____

_____

_____

_____

Today's headline:

_____

_____

One dream I have for my family in five years is...

_____

_____

_____

_____

_____

Right now, in this moment, I am grateful for...

_____

_____

_____

_____

The MOST important thing I can do to feel good about myself today is...

_____

_____

_____

Today, I want to be...

_____

_____

_____

_____

_____

_____

_____

_____

_____

Today, I want to feel...

_____

_____

_____

_____

I am so much stronger than...

_____

_____

_____

_____

Today's headline:

_____

_____

One dream I have for my family in five years is...

_____

_____

_____

_____

_____

Right now, in this moment, I am grateful for...

_____

_____

_____

_____

The MOST important thing I can do to feel good about myself today is...

_____

_____

_____

Today, I want to be...

_____

_____

_____

_____

_____

_____

_____

_____

_____

Today, I want to feel...

_____

_____

_____

_____

I am so much stronger than...

_____

_____

_____

_____

Today's headline:

_____

_____

One dream I have for my family in five years is...

_____

_____

_____

_____

_____

Right now, in this moment, I am grateful for...

_____

_____

_____

_____

The MOST important thing I can do to feel good about myself today is...

_____

_____

_____

Today, I want to be...

_____

_____

_____

_____

_____

_____

_____

_____

_____

Today, I want to feel...

_____

_____

_____

_____

I am so much stronger than...

_____

_____

_____

_____

Today's headline:

_____

_____

One dream I have for my family in five years is...

_____

_____

_____

_____

_____

	Identity	Net Outcome (+ / n / −)	Learnings to take forward
	Reflections (from last week)		
1.			
2.			
3.			
4.			
5.			
6.			
7.			

Right now, in this moment, I am grateful for...

The MOST important thing I can do to feel good about myself today is...

Today, I want to be...

Today, I want to feel...

_____

_____

_____

_____

I am so much stronger than...

_____

_____

_____

_____

Today's headline:

_____

_____

One dream I have for my family in five years is...

_____

_____

_____

_____

_____

Right now, in this moment, I am grateful for...

_____

_____

_____

_____

The MOST important thing I can do to feel good about myself today is...

_____

_____

_____

Today, I want to be...

_____

_____

_____

_____

_____

_____

_____

_____

_____

Today, I want to feel...

_____
_____
_____
_____

I am so much stronger than...

_____
_____
_____
_____

Today's headline:

_____
_____

One dream I have for my family in five years is...

_____
_____
_____
_____
_____

Week 10, Day 3

Right now, in this moment, I am grateful for...

_____

_____

_____

_____

The MOST important thing I can do to feel good about myself today is...

_____

_____

_____

Today, I want to be...

_____

_____

_____

_____

_____

_____

_____

_____

_____

Today, I want to feel...

_____

_____

_____

_____

I am so much stronger than...

_____

_____

_____

_____

Today's headline:

_____

_____

One dream I have for my family in five years is...

_____

_____

_____

_____

_____

Week 10, Day 4

Right now, in this moment, I am grateful for...

_____
_____
_____
_____

The MOST important thing I can do to feel good about myself today is...

_____
_____
_____

Today, I want to be...

_____
_____
_____
_____
_____
_____
_____
_____
_____

Today, I want to feel...

I am so much stronger than...

Today's headline:

One dream I have for my family in five years is...

Week 10, Day 5

Right now, in this moment, I am grateful for...

_____

_____

_____

_____

The MOST important thing I can do to feel good about myself today is...

_____

_____

_____

Today, I want to be...

_____

_____

_____

_____

_____

_____

_____

_____

_____

Today, I want to feel...

I am so much stronger than...

Today's headline:

One dream I have for my family in five years is...

Right now, in this moment, I am grateful for...

_____

_____

_____

_____

The MOST important thing I can do to feel good about myself today is...

_____

_____

_____

Today, I want to be...

_____

_____

_____

_____

_____

_____

_____

_____

_____

Today, I want to feel...

_____

_____

_____

_____

I am so much stronger than...

_____

_____

_____

_____

Today's headline:

_____

_____

One dream I have for my family in five years is...

_____

_____

_____

_____

_____

Right now, in this moment, I am grateful for...

_____

_____

_____

_____

The MOST important thing I can do to feel good about myself today is...

_____

_____

_____

Today, I want to be...

_____

_____

_____

_____

_____

_____

_____

_____

_____

Today, I want to feel...

_____

_____

_____

_____

I am so much stronger than...

_____

_____

_____

_____

Today's headline:

_____

_____

One dream I have for my family in five years is...

_____

_____

_____

_____

_____

	Reflections (from last week)		
	Identity	Net Outcome (+ / n / −)	Learnings to take forward
1.			
2.			
3.			
4.			
5.			
6.			
7.			

Week 11: __ / __ / __

195

Right now, in this moment, I am grateful for...

_____

_____

_____

_____

The MOST important thing I can do to feel good about myself today is...

_____

_____

_____

Today, I want to be...

_____

_____

_____

_____

_____

_____

_____

_____

_____

Today, I want to feel…

_____

_____

_____

_____

I am so much stronger than…

_____

_____

_____

_____

Today's headline:

_____

_____

One dream I have for my family in five years is…

_____

_____

_____

_____

_____

Right now, in this moment, I am grateful for...

The MOST important thing I can do to feel good about myself today is...

Today, I want to be...

Today, I want to feel…

_____

_____

_____

_____

I am so much stronger than…

_____

_____

_____

_____

Today's headline:

_____

_____

One dream I have for my family in five years is…

_____

_____

_____

_____

_____

Right now, in this moment, I am grateful for...

The MOST important thing I can do to feel good about myself today is...

Today, I want to be...

Today, I want to feel...

_____

_____

_____

_____

I am so much stronger than...

_____

_____

_____

_____

Today's headline:

_____

_____

One dream I have for my family in five years is...

_____

_____

_____

_____

_____

Right now, in this moment, I am grateful for...

_____

_____

_____

_____

The MOST important thing I can do to feel good about myself today is...

_____

_____

_____

Today, I want to be...

_____

_____

_____

_____

_____

_____

_____

_____

_____

Today, I want to feel…

_____

_____

_____

_____

I am so much stronger than…

_____

_____

_____

_____

Today's headline:

_____

_____

One dream I have for my family in five years is…

_____

_____

_____

_____

_____

Week 11, Day 5

Right now, in this moment, I am grateful for...

_____
_____
_____
_____

The MOST important thing I can do to feel good about myself today is...

_____
_____
_____

Today, I want to be...

_____
_____
_____
_____
_____
_____
_____
_____
_____

Today, I want to feel...

_____

_____

_____

_____

I am so much stronger than...

_____

_____

_____

_____

Today's headline:

_____

_____

One dream I have for my family in five years is...

_____

_____

_____

_____

_____

Right now, in this moment, I am grateful for...

The MOST important thing I can do to feel good about myself today is...

Today, I want to be...

Today, I want to feel...

_____

_____

_____

_____

I am so much stronger than...

_____

_____

_____

_____

Today's headline:

_____

_____

One dream I have for my family in five years is...

_____

_____

_____

_____

_____

Right now, in this moment, I am grateful for...

_____

_____

_____

_____

The MOST important thing I can do to feel good about myself today is...

_____

_____

_____

Today, I want to be...

_____

_____

_____

_____

_____

_____

_____

_____

_____

Today, I want to feel...

_____

_____

_____

_____

I am so much stronger than...

_____

_____

_____

_____

Today's headline:

_____

_____

One dream I have for my family in five years is...

_____

_____

_____

_____

_____

	Reflections (from last week)		
	Identity	Net Outcome (+ / n / −)	Learnings to take forward
1.			
2.			
3.			
4.			
5.			
6.			
7.			

Right now, in this moment, I am grateful for...

_____

_____

_____

_____

The MOST important thing I can do to feel good about myself today is...

_____

_____

_____

Today, I want to be...

_____

_____

_____

_____

_____

_____

_____

_____

_____

Today, I want to feel…

I am so much stronger than…

Today's headline:

One dream I have for my family in five years is…

Right now, in this moment, I am grateful for...

_____

_____

_____

_____

The MOST important thing I can do to feel good about myself today is...

_____

_____

_____

Today, I want to be...

_____

_____

_____

_____

_____

_____

_____

_____

_____

Today, I want to feel...

_____

_____

_____

_____

I am so much stronger than...

_____

_____

_____

_____

Today's headline:

_____

_____

One dream I have for my family in five years is...

_____

_____

_____

_____

_____

Right now, in this moment, I am grateful for...

The MOST important thing I can do to feel good about myself today is...

Today, I want to be...

Today, I want to feel...

_____

_____

_____

_____

I am so much stronger than...

_____

_____

_____

_____

Today's headline:

_____

_____

One dream I have for my family in five years is...

_____

_____

_____

_____

_____

Right now, in this moment, I am grateful for...

_____

_____

_____

_____

The MOST important thing I can do to feel good about myself today is...

_____

_____

_____

Today, I want to be...

_____

_____

_____

_____

_____

_____

_____

_____

_____

Today, I want to feel…

I am so much stronger than…

Today's headline:

One dream I have for my family in five years is…

Right now, in this moment, I am grateful for...

_____

_____

_____

_____

The MOST important thing I can do to feel good about myself today is...

_____

_____

_____

Today, I want to be...

_____

_____

_____

_____

_____

_____

_____

_____

_____

Today, I want to feel...

_____

_____

_____

_____

I am so much stronger than...

_____

_____

_____

_____

Today's headline:

_____

_____

One dream I have for my family in five years is...

_____

_____

_____

_____

_____

Right now, in this moment, I am grateful for...

_____

_____

_____

_____

The MOST important thing I can do to feel good about myself today is...

_____

_____

_____

Today, I want to be...

_____

_____

_____

_____

_____

_____

_____

_____

_____

_____

Today, I want to feel…

_____

_____

_____

_____

I am so much stronger than…

_____

_____

_____

_____

Today's headline:

_____

_____

One dream I have for my family in five years is…

_____

_____

_____

_____

_____

Right now, in this moment, I am grateful for...

_____

_____

_____

_____

The MOST important thing I can do to feel good about myself today is...

_____

_____

_____

Today, I want to be...

_____

_____

_____

_____

_____

_____

_____

_____

_____

Today, I want to feel...

_____

_____

_____

_____

I am so much stronger than...

_____

_____

_____

_____

Today's headline:

_____

_____

One dream I have for my family in five years is...

_____

_____

_____

_____

_____

A FINAL VISION FOR OUR CHILDREN

What if our children learned...
To count numbers AND blessings
To exercise muscles AND compassion
To write essays AND letters of encouragement
To design 3D models AND their best lives
To locate Hawaii AND their true self
To feel smart AND loved
Let's start there.
Because that is where dreams are given flight.
That is where change begins.
That is what our future world needs.

Good luck momma! You've got this.

With all the love & support I have to give,

Lisa Colella

CPSIA information can be obtained
at www.ICGtesting.com
Printed in the USA
BVHW050145051120
592523BV00002B/10